Copyright © 2020 by Patricia James MD

All rights reserved. No part of this publication may be reproduced, distributed, or transmitted in any form or by any means, including photocopying, recording, or other electronic or mechanical methods, without the prior written permission of the publisher, except in the case of brief quotations embodied in critical reviews and certain other noncommercial uses permitted by copyright law

Table of Contents

Introduction...5

    What is Pancreatitis?...5

Causes of pancreatitis 7

How can foods affect your pancreas? 8

    Nutrition treatment for pancreatitis.................................9

Pancreatitis Diet...11

    Foods to include in a pancreatitis diet 14

    Foods to avoid in a pancreatitis diet..............................15

Choosing a Pancreatitis Diet**Error! Bookmark not defined.**

General Recipe Substitutions for People with Pancreatitis ....**Error! Bookmark not defined.**

Diet Tips for People with Pancreatitis**Error! Bookmark not defined.**

7-Day Pancreatitis Diet Meal Plan.......................................16

    Pancreatitis Diet Sample Menu**Error! Bookmark not defined.**

Pancreatitis Diet Recipes 36

    Breakfast 36

        Banana Blueberry Muffins 45

Baked Berry French Toast 46

Apple Butternut Squash Pancakes 48

Apple and Oat Bake 50

Summer Vegetables Omelet 52

Pancakes 36

Steel Cut Oats with Cranberries and Walnuts 37

Apple Banana Smoothie 39

Spinach and Cheese Frittata 41

Baked Broccoli Frittata 43

Lunch and Dinner 54

Asparagus Frittata 65

Edamame Hummus Wrap 67

Chicken Salad Sandwich 68

Hearty Vegetable and Lentil Soup 70

Pastiera (Pasta Egg Bake) 72

Chicken with Quinoa 54

Turkey Meatloaf (Mini) 55

Turkey Tortellini Soup 57

Shrimp Pomodoro & Angel Hair 61

Apps & Sides 74

Maple Green Beans 74

Carrot Purée with Olive Oil and Cilantro 75

Vegetable Popover 77

Butternut Squash Soup 79

Desserts & Beverages 97

Rice Pudding 97

Peaches and Cream Smoothie 99

Grilled Pineapple 101

Banana Peach Sorbet 102

Baked Apples 103

Holiday & Seasonal Ideas 81

Chicken Kebab with Tzatziki and Pita 81

Pumpkin Oatmeal Bars 83

Sweet Potato and White Bean Fritters 86

Thanksgiving Meatballs 88

Sole En Papillote with Citrus and Ginger 90

Vegan Tofu Lasagna 92

Turkey Sweet Potato Hash 94

The Bottom Line 105

Introduction

The Pancreas is an organ that sits behind the stomach and plays an important role in digesting food and regulating blood sugar.

Pancreatitis is a serious problem that can disrupt the normal function of the pancreas and may require changes to the way you eat.

This book will provide an overview of pancreatitis and how to manage this condition from a nutrition point of view.

What is Pancreatitis?

Pancreatitis is an inflammation of the pancreas, and it occurs when the pancreas attacks itself with the same digestive enzymes that are normally used to break down food.

Pancreatitis comes in two main types: acute and chronic. For those at risk of pancreatitis, A doctor may use a special test known as an endoscopic retrograde cholangiopancreatography (ERCP) to diagnosis the exact issues.

Acute pancreatitis: Pancreatitis that appears suddenly is known as acute pancreatitis. Symptoms include:

- severe abdominal pain
- nausea
- vomiting
- rapid heart rate

Acute pancreatitis usually resolves quickly with proper treatment, which may include hospitalization for IV fluids, medication to manage pain, and giving your stomach a rest. In some cases, acute pancreatitis can be life-threatening, and any symptoms should be taken seriously.

Chronic pancreatitis: When the pancreas is permanently damaged from inflammation, the condition becomes long-lasting, as is known as chronic pancreatitis. Chronic pancreatitis usually develops slowly over time and can diminish your ability to digest food (this is known as the pancreatic exocrine deficiency). Symptoms people with pancreatitis may experience include:

- diarrhea

- fatty stools
- abdominal pain – especially with fatty foods
- unintentional weight loss
- formation of a painful cyst known as a pancreatic pseudocyst.

There is no cure for chronic pancreatitis, but the condition can be managed, and the damage can be slowed. Treatment usually involves the correct diet, taking pancreatic enzymes, and managing symptoms.

Causes of pancreatitis

The most common cause of pancreatitis is gallstones. Gallstones are an abnormal buildup of bile, a substance that is stored in the gallbladder.

Sometimes, these gallstones can block the pancreas from releasing digestive enzymes. These blocked enzymes then start to eat and damage the pancreas itself, a process called autodigestion.

The next most common cause is excessive alcohol consumption. Alcohol is partially metabolized in the pancreas and produces byproducts that are toxic in large quantities.

Researchers are still working to understand exactly why some people with alcoholism get pancreatitis while most do not.

Other causes of pancreatitis include:

- Genetic factors
- Certain medications
- Abdominal trauma
- Infection
- Cancer
- Cystic fibrosis

How can foods affect your pancreas?

To break down the foods you eat, your pancreas secretes three different kinds of digestive enzymes: protease, amylin, and lipase, which break down proteins, sugars, and fats, respectively.

Thus, eating a heavy meal such as a greasy pizza will activate the pancreas to release a large number of enzymes to fully break down the food.

The pizza will also contain many carbohydrates, which will require the pancreas to release insulin to regulate the blood sugar response to the meal.

Nutrition treatment for pancreatitis

Because the pancreas is very involved with handling meals, nutrition plays an important role in the treatment of pancreatitis.

For acute pancreatitis, the focus is on giving the pancreas time to rest. This may involve a period of fasting with nothing but fluids for a little while.

As symptoms improve, you may progress to a diet that is low in fat and concentrated sugars to reduce the burden on the pancreas. Since acute pancreatitis lasts only a short while, this may be all that is required to manage the condition.

In those that are at risk for malnutrition, tube feeding is sometimes used to supply carefully tailored nutrition without harming the pancreas.

In rare cases, when all forms of food are not tolerated for an extended period, intravenous nutrition (known as parenteral nutrition) is needed.

Nutrition is a significant part of the lifestyle of people with chronic pancreatitis. Since the damage done in chronic pancreatitis cannot be reversed, eating right can help to slow down the damage and keep the pancreas working as well as possible.

There are several priorities for nutrition management in chronic pancreatitis:

- **Preventing malnutrition.** The risk of nutrient deficiencies is high due to reduced absorption from food, lower appetite, pain with eating, and increased energy needs from inflammation.
- **Reducing strain on the pancreas.** The pancreas will work harder and produce more digestive enzymes in heavy meals, especially those high in fats and sugars. Keeping these nutrients in moderation (but not eliminating them) is important to reduce pancreatic inflammation. If pancreatic enzymes are needed, these should be taken will all meals and snacks to assist the pancreas with digestion.
- **Controlling blood sugar.** Remember that a damaged pancreas may not be able to keep up with the blood sugar demands of the body. To help it out,

making certain diet changes, especially with portion control and carbohydrate moderation, can help keep sugars in check.
- **Avoiding alcohol.** Alcohol abuse can cause immediate discomfort in pancreatitis and will further exacerbate the condition. It is best to avoid alcohol entirely with pancreatitis.

With these priorities in mind, what does a pancreatitis diet actually look like?

Pancreatitis Diet

A pancreatitis diet includes the following components:

- **Small, frequent meals.** Spreading out meals into smaller chunks is usually better tolerated as they are easier for the pancreas to handle. Eating frequently also helps to prevent malnutrition. Aim for about 6 meals per day.
- **Moderate to low fat.** You will want to keep total fat to about 30% of total calories. This includes all types of fat, even healthier fats such as olive oil. It may be a good idea to log all meals for a few days into a nutrition

analyzing software such as the USDA nutrient database to get a feel for how much total fat you usually eat.

- **Consider MCT oil.** MCT stands for medium-chain triglycerides, which is a type of fat that does not require pancreatic enzymes to be absorbed. Some evidence suggests that these oils can be better tolerated, and can improve diarrhea associated with pancreatitis. MCT can be taken in supplement form.
- **High-quality lean protein.** Protein is important for healing and maintaining strength. Since many protein sources also contain fat, it is essential to prioritize lean protein choices such as turkey, fish, chicken, or plant sources.
- **Plenty of fruits and vegetables.** Try to make half of your plate fruits and vegetables. This will ensure that vitamin and mineral needs are being met. They also contain antioxidants, phytochemicals, and other beneficial compounds to fight inflammation. Fruits and vegetables also contain fiber, which will help keep to control spikes in blood sugar.
- **Less Processed foods.** Processed foods are generally low in fiber, high in sugars, fat, and sodium and of poor nutrient quality. Choosing whole, unprocessed foods,

whenever possible, is a key part of the pancreatitis diet.

- **Choose the right types and amounts of Carbohydrates.** Carbohydrates (sugars and starches) are an essential energy source, and they generally should make up about 50% of the total calories. However, not all carbohydrates are created equal. Whole grains are preferred to their higher fiber and nutrient content.
- **Avoid too much-added sugar.** Added sugars are sugars not naturally present in a food item; they can make it very easy to have too much sugar without realizing it. Added sugars are found in sodas, sports drinks, juices, candy, pastries, and many other foods. Check the nutrition facts label for the most accurate information.
- **Adequate fluids.** Staying hydrated is a commonly overlooked aspect of nutrition, but it is no less important. About 8-10 cups of fluid per day are recommended. If you have trouble getting enough fluid, consider keeping a refillable water bottle with you as a reminder.

Foods to include in a pancreatitis diet

The following are examples of foods for pancreatitis:

Fruits and vegetables: Apple, Blueberries, Raspberries, Orange, Banana, Spinach, Cauliflower, Broccoli, Tomato, Green Beans

Most fruits and vegetables can be included in a pancreatitis diet plan and will be well tolerated. An exception is a grapefruit, which can interact with many medications. Ask your doctor about grapefruit if you eat it regularly.

Starches: Potato, Sweet Potato, Brown rice, Whole wheat bread, Whole wheat pasta, Black beans, Oatmeal, Corn.

Meats/proteins: Skinless chicken breast, Skinless turkey breast, Fish, Egg whites, Whole egg (1-2 per day), Tofu, Protein powder.

Fats (limit overall fat): Olive oil, Oil sprays, MCT oil, Almonds, Cashews, Peanuts, Walnuts, Seeds, low-fat cottage cheese

Beverages: Water, Skim or 1% milk, Sugar-free seltzer water.

Foods to avoid in a pancreatitis diet

Keep the following foods limited as much as possible. Keep in mind that this list is not comprehensive, and you should use the above priorities to guide your eating choices.

- Sausages
- Processed meats such as salami, pepperoni, and roast beef.
- High-fat red meats such as ribeye steak and burgers.
- Fried foods, including french fries.
- Processed, high-fat cheeses such as American and cheddar.
- Bacon, Butter, Cream soups, Whole milk, Ice-cream, Candy, Soda, Juice, Sports drinks, Alcohol, Sugary cereal, Chocolate, Avocado.

One Week Pancreatitis Diet Meal Plan

Day 1: Monday

Breakfast: Banana Yogurt Pots

Nutrition: Calories – 236, Protein – 14g, Carbs – 32g, Fat – 7g

Prep time: 5 minutes

Ingredients (for 2 people)

- 225g Greek yogurt
- 2 bananas, sliced into chunks
- 15g walnuts, toasted and chopped

Instructions

1. Place some of the yogurt into the bottom of a glass. Add a layer of banana, then yogurt and repeat. Once the glass is full, scatter with the nuts.

Lunch: Cannellini Bean Salad

Nutrition: Calories – 302, Protein – 20g, Carbs – 54g, Fat – 0g

Prep time: 5 minutes

Ingredients (for 2 people)

- 600g cans cannellini beans
- 70g cherry tomatoes, halved
- ½ red onion, thinly sliced
- ½ tbsp red wine vinegar
- small bunch basil, torn

Instructions

1. Rinse and drain the beans and mix with the tomatoes, onion and vinegar. Season, then add basil just before serving.

Dinner: Quick'n'Easy Moussaka

Nutrition: Calories – 577 Protein – 27g Carbs – 46g Fat – 27g

Prep time + cook time: 30 minutes

Ingredients (for 2 people)

- 1 tbsp extra virgin olive oil

- ½ onion, finely chopped
- 1 garlic clove, finely chopped
- 250g lean beef mince
- 200g can chopped tomatoes
- 1 tbsp tomato purée
- 1 tsp ground cinnamon
- 200g can chickpeas
- 100g pack feta cheese, crumbled
- Mint (fresh preferable)
- Brown bread, to serve

Instructions

1. Heat the oil in a pan. Add the onion and garlic and fry until soft. Add the mince and fry for 3-4 minutes until browned.
2. Tip the tomatoes into the pan and stir in the tomato purée and cinnamon, then season. Leave the mince to simmer for 20 minutes. Add the chickpeas halfway through.
3. Sprinkle the feta and mint over the mince. Serve with toasted bread.

Day 2: Tuesday

Breakfast: Tomato and Watermelon Salad

Nutrition: Calories – 177 Protein – 5g Carbs – 13g Fat – 13g

Prep time + cook time: 5 minutes

Ingredients (for 2 people)

- 1 tbsp olive oil
- 1 tbsp red wine vinegar
- ¼ tsp chilli flakes
- 1 tbsp chopped mint
- 120g tomatoes, chopped
- 250g watermelon, cut into chunks
- 50g feta cheese, crumbled

Instructions

1. For the dressing, Mix the oil, vinegar, chilli flakes and mint and then season.

2. Put the tomatoes and watermelon into a bowl. Pour over the dressing, add the feta, then serve.

Lunch: Edgy Veggie Wraps

Nutrition: Calories – 310 Protein – 11g Carbs – 39g Fat – 11g

Prep time + cook time: 10 minutes

Ingredients (for 2 people)

- 100g cherry tomatoes
- 1 cucumber
- 6 Kalamata olives
- 2 large wholemeal tortilla wraps
- 50g feta cheese
- 2 tbsp houmous

Instructions

1. Chop the tomatoes, cut the cucumber into sticks, split the olives and remove the stones.

2. Heat the tortillas.

3. Spread the houmous over the wrap. Put the vegetable mix in the middle and roll up.

Dinner: Spicy Tomato Baked Eggs

Nutrition: Calories – 417 Protein – 19g Carbs – 45g Fat – 17g

Prep time + cook time: 25 minutes

Ingredients (for 2 people)

- 1 tbsp olive oil
- 2 red onions, chopped
- 1 red chilli, deseeded & chopped
- 1 garlic clove, sliced
- small bunch coriander, stalks and leaves chopped separately
- 800g can cherry tomatoes
- 4 eggs
- brown bread, to serve

Instructions

1. Heat the oil in a frying pan with a lid, then cook the onions, chilli, garlic and coriander stalks for 5 minutes until soft. Stir in the tomatoes, then simmer for 8-10 minutes.

2. Using the back of a large spoon, make 4 dips in the sauce, then crack an egg into each one. Put a lid on the pan, then

cook over a low heat for 6-8 mins, until the eggs are done to your liking. Scatter with the coriander leaves and serve with bread.

Day 3: Wednesday

Breakfast: Blueberry Oats Bowl

Nutrition: Calories – 235 Protein – 13g Carbs – 38g Fat – 4g

Prep time + cook time: 10 minutes

Ingredients (for 2 people)

- 60g porridge oats
- 160g Greek yogurt
- 175g blueberries
- 1 tsp honey

Instructions

1. Put the oats in a pan with 400ml of water. Heat and stir for about 2 minutes. Remove from the heat and add a third of the yogurt.

2. Tip the blueberries into a pan with the honey and 1 tbsp of water. Gently poach until the blueberries are tender.

3. Spoon the porridge into bowls and add the remaining yogurt and blueberries.

Lunch: Carrot, Orange and Avocado Salad

Nutrition: Calories – 177 Protein – 5g Carbs – 13g Fat – 13g

Prep time + cook time: 5 minutes

Ingredients (for 2 people)

- 1 orange, plus zest and juice of 1
- 2 carrots, halved lengthways and sliced with a peeler
- 35g bag rocket/arugala
- 1 avocado, stoned, peeled and sliced
- 1 tbsp olive oil

Instructions

1. Cut the segments from 1 of the oranges and put in a bowl with the carrots, rocket and avocado. Whisk together the orange juice, zest and oil. Toss through the salad, and season.

Dinner: Salmon with Potatoes and Corn Salad

Nutrition: Calories – 479 Protein – 43g Carbs – 27g Fat – 21g

Prep time + cook time: 30 minutes

Ingredients (for 2 people)

- 200g baby new potatoes
- 1 sweetcorn cob
- 2 skinless salmon fillets
- 60g tomatoes
- 1 tbsp red wine vinegar
- 1 tbsp extra-virgin olive oil
- 1 shallot, finely chopped
- 1 tbsp capers, finely chopped
- handful basil leaves

Instructions

1. Cook potatoes in boiling water until tender, adding corn for final 5 minutes. Drain & cool.

2. For the dressing, mix the vinegar, oil, shallot, capers, basil & seasoning.

3. Heat grill to high. Rub some dressing on salmon & cook, skinnedside down, for 7-8 minutes. Slice tomatoes & place on plate. Slice the potatoes, cut the corn from the cob & add to plate. Add the salmon & drizzle over the remaining dressing.

Day 4: Thursday

Breakfast: Banana Yogurt Pots

Lunch: Mixed Bean Salad

Nutrition Calories – 240 Protein – 11g Carbs – 22g Fat – 12g

Prep time + cook time: 10 minutes

Ingredients (for 2 people)

- 145g jar artichoke heart in oil
- ½ tbsp sundried tomato paste
- ½ tsp red wine vinegar
- 200g can cannellini beans, drained and rinsed
- 150g pack tomatoes, quartered handful Kalamata black olives
- 2 spring onions, thinly sliced on the diagonal
- 100g feta cheese, crumbled

Instructions

1. Drain the jar of artichokes, reserving 1-2 tbsp of oil. Add the oil, sun-dried tomato paste and vinegar and stir until smooth. Season to taste.

2. Chop the artichokes and tip into a bowl. Add the cannellini beans, tomatoes, olives, spring onions and half of the feta cheese. Stir in the artichoke oil mixture and tip into a serving bowl. Crumble over the remaining feta cheese, then serve.

Dinner: Spiced Carrot and Lentil Soup

Nutrition: Calories – 238 Protein – 11g Carbs – 34g Fat – 7g

Prep time + cook time: 25 minutes

Ingredients (for 2 people)

- 1 tsp cumin seeds
- pinch chilli flakes
- 1 tbsp olive oil
- 300g carrots, washed and coarsely grated (no need to peel)
- 70g split red lentils

- 500ml hot vegetable stock (from a cube is fine)
- 60ml milk
- Greek yogurt, to serve

Instructions

1. Heat a large saucepan and dry fry the cumin seeds and chilli flakes for 1 minute. Scoop out about half of the seeds with a spoon and set aside. Add the oil, carrot, lentils, stock and milk to the pan and bring to the boil. Simmer for 15 minutes until the lentils have swollen and softened.

2. Whizz the soup with a stick blender or in a food processor until smooth. Season to taste and finish with a dollop of Greek yogurt and a sprinkling of the reserved toasted spices.

Day 5: Friday

Breakfast: Tomato and Watermelon Salad

Lunch: Panzanella Salad

Nutrition: Calories – 452 Protein – 6g Carbs – 37g Fat – 25g

Prep time + cook time: 10 minutes

Ingredients (for 2 people)

- 400g tomatoes
- 1 garlic clove, crushed
- 1 tbsp capers, drained and rinsed
- 1 ripe avocado, stoned, peeled and chopped
- 1 small red onion, very thinly sliced
- 2 slices of brown bread
- 2 tbsp olive oil
- 1 tbsp red wine vinegar
- small handful basil leaves

Instructions

1. Chop the tomatoes and put them in a bowl. Season well and add the garlic, capers, avocado and onion. Mix well and set aside for 10 minutes.

2. Meanwhile, tear the bread into chunks and place in a bowl. Drizzle over half of the olive oil and half of the vinegar. When ready to serve, scatter tomatoes and basil leaves and drizzle with remaining oil and vinegar. Stir before serving.

Dinner: Med Chicken, Quinoa and Greek Salad

Nutrition: Calories – 473 Protein – 36g Carbs – 57g Fat – 25g

Prep time + cook time: 20 minutes

Ingredients (for 2 people)

- 100g quinoa
- ½ red chilli, deseeded and finely chopped
- 1 garlic clove, crushed
- 200g chicken
- 1 tbsp extra-virgin olive oil
- 150g tomato, roughly chopped
- handful pitted black kalamata olives
- ½ red onion, finely sliced
- 50g feta cheese, crumbled
- small bunch mint leaves, chopped
- juice and zest ½ lemon

Instructions

1. Cook the quinoa following the pack instructions, then rinse in cold water and drain thoroughly.

2. Meanwhile, toss the chicken fillets in the olive oil with some seasoning, chilli and garlic. Lay in a hot pan and cook for 3-4 minutes each side or until cooked through. Transfer to a plate and set aside

3. Next, tip the tomatoes, olives, onion, feta and mint into a bowl. Toss in the cooked quinoa. Stir through the remaining olive oil, lemon juice and zest, and season well. Serve with the chicken on top.

Day 6: Saturday

Breakfast: Blueberry Oats Bowl

Lunch: Quinoa and Stir Fried Veg

Nutrition: Calories – 473 Protein – 11g Carbs – 56g Fat – 25g

Prep time + cook time: 30 minutes

Ingredients (for 2 people)

- 100g quinoa
- 3 tbsp olive oil

- 1 garlic clove, finely chopped
- 2 carrots, cut into thin sticks
- 150g leek, sliced
- 150g broccoli, cut into small florets
- 50g tomatoes
- 100ml vegetable stock
- 1 tsp tomato purée
- juice ½ lemon

Instructions

1. Cook the quinoa according to pack instructions. Meanwhile, heat 3 tbsp of the oil in a pan, then add the garlic and quickly fry for 1 minute. Throw in the carrots, leeks and broccoli, then stir-fry for 2 minutes until everything is glistening.

2. Add the tomatoes, mix together the stock and tomato purée, then add to the pan. Cover and cook for 3 minutes. Drain the quinoa and toss in the remaining oil and lemon juice. Divide between warm plates and spoon the vegetables on top.

Dinner: Grilled Vegetables with Bean Mash

Nutrition: Calories – 314 Protein – 19g Carbs – 33g Fat – 16g

Prep time + cook time: 40 minutes

Ingredients (for 2 people)

- 1 tbsp olive oil
- 1 tbsp red wine vinegar
- ¼ tsp chilli flakes
- 1 tbsp chopped mint
- 120g tomatoes, chopped
- 250g watermelon, cut into chunks
- 50g feta cheese, crumbled

Instructions

1. Heat the grill. Arrange the vegetables over a grill pan & brush lightly with oil. Grill until lightly browned, turn them over, brush again with oil, then grill until tender.

2. Meanwhile, put the beans in a pan with garlic and stock. Bring to the boil, then simmer, uncovered, for 10 minutes. Mash roughly with a potato masher. Divide the vegetables and mash between 2 plates, drizzle over oil and sprinkle with black pepper and coriander.

Day 7: Sunday

Breakfast: Banana Yogurt Pots

Lunch: Moroccan Chickpea Soup

Nutrition: Calories – 408 Protein – 15g Carbs – 63g Fat – 11g

Prep time + cook time: 25 minutes

Ingredients (for 2 people)

- 1 tbsp olive oil
- ½ medium onion, chopped
- 1 celery sticks, chopped
- 1 tsp ground cumin
- 300ml hot vegetable stock
- 200g can chopped tomatoes
- 200g can chickpeas, rinsed and drained
- 50g frozen broad beans
- zest and juice ½ lemon
- coriander & bread to serve

Instructions

1. Heat the oil in a saucepan, then fry the onion and celery for 10 minutes until softened. Add the cumin and fry for another minute.

2. Turn up the heat, then add the stock, tomatoes, chickpeas and black pepper. Simmer for 8 minutes. Add broad beans and lemon juice and cook for a further 2 minutes. Top with lemon zest and coriander.

Dinner: Spicy Mediterranean Beet Salad

Nutrition: Calories – 548 Protein – 23g Carbs – 58g Fat – 20g

Prep time + cook time: 40 minutes

Ingredients (for 2 people)

- 8 raw baby beetroots, or 4 medium, scrubbed
- ½ tbsp za'atar
- ½ tbsp sumac
- ½ tbsp ground cumin
- 400g can chickpeas, drained and rinsed
- 2 tbsp olive oil

- ½ tsp lemon zest
- ½ tsp lemon juice
- 200g Greek yogurt
- 1 tbsp harissa paste
- 1 tsp crushed red chilli flakes
- mint leaves, chopped, to serve

Instructions

1. Heat oven to 220C/200C fan/ gas 7. Halve or quarter beetroots depending on size. Mix spices together. On a large baking tray, mix chickpeas and beetroot with the oil. Season with salt & sprinkle over the spices. Mix again. Roast for 30 minutes.

2. While the vegetables are cooking, mix the lemon zest and juice with the yogurt. Swirl the harissa through and spread into a bowl. Top with the beetroot & chickpeas, and sprinkle with the chilli flakes & mint.

Pancreatitis Diet Recipes

Breakfast

Pancakes

If you're watching your fat intake, these lower fat pancakes are perfect and if you're not, it's fine to add a bit of unsalted butter. Either way, top with real maple syrup: don't consider using the fake stuff.

Makes about 12 6- inch pancakes (one pancake)

Ingredients

- 1 1/2 cups all purpose white flour
- ¼ cup whole wheat graham flour 1/4 cup yellow cornmeal
- 1 tablespoon white sugar 1 teaspoon baking soda
- 2 teaspoons baking powder 1/2 teaspoon kosher salt
- 2 cups skim milk buttermilk 1/2 cup skim milk
- 1 large egg
- 2 large egg whites
- 1 tablespoon melted unsalted butter or canola oil

Directions

1. Place the flours, cornmeal, sugar, baking soda, baking powder and salt in a large bowl and stir to combine.
2. Place the buttermilk, skim milk, egg, egg whites and butter in a small bowl and stir to combine. Add the wet ingredients to the dry ingredients and mix until just combined. Do not over- mix.
3. Place a large non- stick skillet over a medium heat and when it is hot, drop ladlefuls of batter on the surface. Cook until bubbles form. Flip over and cook for about 2 minutes. Serve immediately with real maple syrup.

Nutritional Information:

Calories 121, Total Fat 2g, Saturated Fat 1g, Trans Fat 0g, Cholesterol 56 mg, Sodium 268mg, Total Carbohydrates 20g, Dietary Fiber 1g, Protein 5g

Steel Cut Oats with Cranberries and Walnuts

There is no question that steel cut oats are far better – in flavor, texture and taste- than rolled oats. However, the common complaint- that they take forever to cook- is a fair one. My solution: start the process the night before!

This recipe serves one but can easily be quadrupled. Serves one

Ingredients

- 1/3 cup steel cut oats 1 1/3 cup water
- To each serving add:
- 2 tablespoons skim milk
- 1 tablespoon dried cranberries, raisins, dates, apricots or cherries
- 1 teaspoon lightly toasted chopped walnuts, pecans or almonds (optional) 1 teaspoon ground flax seed (optional)
- ½ teaspoon wheat bran
- 1 teaspoon maple syrup, brown sugar or honey Other options, per serving:
- apples and cinnamon sugar blueberries

Directions

1. The night before: Place the oatmeal and water in a small saucepan and bring to a boil over high heat. Cover and cool to room temperature. Refrigerate overnight.

2. The next morning: Remove the cover, place the saucepan over high heat and bring to a boil. Reduce the heat to low, partially cover and cook until the oatmeal is tender, 10- 15 minutes. Add the milk, cranberries, nuts, flax, wheat and maple syrup, as desired. Serve immediately.

Nutritional Information:

With Flax Seed: Calories 272, Total Fat 6g, Saturated Fat 1g, Trans Fat 0g, Cholesterol 0mg, Sodium 19mg, Total Carbohydrates 44g, Dietary Fibers 11g, Protein 11g

Without Flax Seed: Calories 255, Total Fat 5g, Saturated Fat 1g, Trans Fat 0g, Cholesterol 1mg, Sodium 26mg, Total Carbohydrate 43g, Dietary Fiber 6g, Protein 10g

Apple Banana Smoothie

Smoothies are infinitely adaptable but here is my basic and most favored version. Feel free to substitute peaches or pears for the apple, and apple or pineapple juice for the orange. I always use bananas; they are indispensable for the smooth texture and creamy mouth-feel they impart. Add nuts or ground flax seed if your diet allows.

Serves 2 (one serving)

Ingredients

- 1 over-ripe banana, cut in 4
- 1 Granny Smith apple, cored and chopped 1 cup non-fat plain yogurt
- 1/2 cup orange juice
- ½ cup water
- 1 tablespoon wheat germ or wheat bran 1 tablespoon ground flax seed (optional)

Ingredients

1. Place the banana and apple in a blender or the bowl of a food processor fitted with a steel blade and process until almost smooth.
2. Add the remaining ingredients and process until smooth.
3. Serve immediately or refrigerate up to one hour.

Nutritional Data:

Smoothie with Flax Seed: Calories 228, Total Fat 2g, Saturated Fat 0g, Trans Fat 0g, Cholesterol 1mg, Sodium 38mg, Total Carbohydrate 50g, Dietary Fiber 5g, Protein 5g

Smoothie without Flax Seed: Calories 209, Total Fat 1g, Saturated Fat 0g, Trans Fat 0g, Cholesterol 1mg, Sodium 37mg, Total Carbohydrate 49g, Dietary Fiber 4g, Protein 5g.

Spinach and Cheese Frittata

The frittata, an open-faced omelet, is one of my favorite dishes: easy to make, infinitely adaptable, full of protein and great for breakfast, brunch, lunch and even a light dinner.

Serves 6 (one serving)

Ingredients

- 1 teaspoon vegetable or olive oil 1 large Spanish onion, chopped 2 garlic cloves, minced
- 6 large eggs, lightly beaten
- 10 large egg whites, lightly beaten
- 2 cups tightly packed flat leaf spinach, chopped or baby spinach, well washed 1/2 cup crumbled non-fat feta cheese or goat cheese
- 1 teaspoon kosher salt
- ½ teaspoon black pepper

Directions

1. Place a non-stick skillet over medium heat and when it is hot, add the oil. Add the onion and garlic and cook, stirring occasionally, until they are fragrant, soft and slightly caramelized, about 8- 12 minutes (depending on the size of the pan). Set aside to cool.
2. Add the remaining ingredients and mix well. The mixture will look very spinach-y and not very egg-y. (The frittata can be completed up to this point the night before. Simply cover and refrigerate).
3. Preheat the oven to 350 degrees. Place a lightly buttered non stick 9 inch square pan in the oven and when both are hot, add the egg mixture and let cook until the eggs are set, 15- 20 minutes.
4. Serve hot, room temp or cold with a little bit of fruit salad on the side or Mesclun greens.

Nutritional Data: Calories 131, Total Fat 6g, Saturated Fat 2g, Trans Fat 0g, Cholesterol 211 mg, Sodium 352 mg, Total Carbohydrate 4g, Dietary Fiber 1g, Protein 13g

Baked Broccoli Frittata

Frittatas are a perfect meal. Good for kids and adults, they can be whipped up in minutes and served hot, cold or at room temperature. They can be filled with just about anything: herbs, vegetables, meats and/or cheeses.

Serves 4

Ingredients

1. 2 teaspoons olive or canola oil
2. 1 small Spanish or purple onion, coarsely chopped 2 garlic cloves, finely chopped
3. 3 cups chopped broccoli florets or zucchini 4 large eggs, lightly beaten
4. 4 large egg whites, lightly beaten 1 cup grated cheese (optional)
5. 1 cup non- fat sour cream, yogurt or ricotta cheese
6. 2 cups cubed day old bread, diced and cooked potatoes or leftover pasta 2 teaspoons kosher salt
7. Preheat the oven to 350 degrees. Lightly grease an 8 inch springform pan or 10-inch pie plate.
8. Place a small pan over a medium low flame and when it is hot, add the oil. Add the onion and garlic and cook until the onion is translucent, about 10 minutes. Add the

broccoli and cook until soft, about 10 minutes. Set aside to cool slightly.

9. Place the remaining ingredients in a mixing bowl and mix, by hand; add the cooled broccoli mixture. The frittata can be completed up to this point the night before. Simply cover and refrigerate.
10. Preheat the oven to 350 degrees.
11. Place a lightly buttered non stick 9-inch square pan in the oven and when both are hot, add the egg mixture and let cook until the eggs are set, 15- 20 minutes.
12. Serve as is or with salsa.

Nutritional Data (with non-fat sour cream): Calories 304, Total Fat 10g, Saturated Fat 2g, Trans Fat 1g, Cholesterol 212mg, Sodium 1052mg, Total Carbohydrate 37g, Dietary Fiber 4g, Protein 19g

Banana Blueberry Muffins

These muffins are a great, quick breakfast treat with bananas and blueberries providing soluble fiber, potassium, and phytonutrients. Non-dairy milk can be substituted for those who are intolerant to lactose and whole-wheat flour can be substituted to increase the fiber content. Yield: 12 muffins

Ingredients:

- 1/2 cup mashed ripe banana (about 1 large)
- 1/2 cup granulated sugar
- 1/2 cup milk (may also sub any non-dairy milk)
- 1/3 cup canola oil
- 1 Tbsp. vanilla extract
- 1 tsp. cinnamon
- 1 cup all-purpose flour (or whole wheat flour)
- 2 tsp. baking powder
- 1/2 cup frozen blueberries

Directions:

1. Preheat oven to 400°F.

2. Line muffin pan with paper cups.

3. In a large bowl, mash the banana with a fork.

4. Add the sugar, milk, oil, vanilla, cinnamon, and whisk until combined.

5. Add the flour, baking powder, and stir until just combined; don't over mix.

6. Fold in 1/2 cup frozen blueberries.

7. Add batter to muffin tin (for easy distribution use medium cookie scoop)

8. Bake for 15-20 minutes, or until tops are slightly golden.

Nutritional Data:

125 calories, 6.4 grams fat, 0.6 grams saturated fat, 1 mg cholesterol, 15.5 grams carbohydrate, 0.7 grams dietary fiber, 1.5 grams protein

Baked Berry French Toast

This French toast recipe is great to make ahead of time for a busy weekday morning. It is a good balanced entrée that includes protein, carbohydrates, dairy, and fruit. Cream cheese and milk components can be substituted with lactose-free versions for those experiencing lactose intolerance.

Yield: 8 Servings

Ingredients:

- 12 slices day-old bread, cut into 1-inch cubes
- 1 (12 oz.) package of low-fat cream cheese, room temperature
- 2 1/4 cups low-fat, fat-free milk, or non-dairy alternative, divided
- 2 tsp. vanilla, divided
- 2 cups blueberries, fresh or thawed frozen, divided
- 10 eggs, beaten
- 1/4 cup plus 1 Tbsp. honey or pure maple syrup

Directions:

1. Preheat oven to 350°F.
2. Lightly grease a 9"x13" inch-baking dish.
3. Blend 1 brick of cream cheese, 1/4 cup of milk, 1 Tbsp. honey and 1 tsp. vanilla.
4. Arrange 1/2 of the bread cubes in bottom of dish. Top with cream cheese mixture. Sprinkle 1 cup of

blueberries over top, and top with remaining bread cubes.

5. In large bowl, mix eggs, milk, vanilla extract, and honey or syrup. Pour over bread cubes Cover, refrigerate 1-hour or overnight.
6. Cover, and bake for 30 minutes. Uncover, and continue baking for 25-30 minutes, until center is firm and surface is lightly browned.
7. Let cool for 10-12 minutes. Top with remaining berries and enjoy.

Nutritional Data: 231 calories, 7.5 grams fat, 1.7 grams saturated fat, 205 mg cholesterol, 29 grams carbohydrate, 3.8 grams dietary fiber, 13.7 grams protein

Apple Butternut Squash Pancakes

These delicious pancakes can be used as a meal any time of the day. They are rich in beta-carotene and are designed to be easy to tolerate for pancreatitis symptoms such as nausea and overall stomach upset. For additional protein, nuts can be added. For those who are experiencing fat intolerance, reduced-fat versions of the dairy components can be substituted, along with lower lactose alternatives for those with lactose intolerance. For those on more severe fiber restrictions, the apple and squash components also can be peeled and boiled to help break down some of the fibers for optimal digestive tolerance. These can be easily frozen (with layers of parchment paper in between) and reheated in the toaster oven or microwave.

Yield: 12 small pancakes (6 large)

Ingredients:

- 3 cups grated raw butternut squash or acorn squash (may also use zucchini)
- 1 large green apple (or 2 small) grated, raw
- 1/3 cup sour cream (use reduced-fat or vegan sour cream if necessary)
- 1 egg
- 1/4 cup milk of choice (use lactose-free, non-dairy, or reduced-fat as needed)
- 1 cup all-purpose flour
- 1 tsp. baking powder

- 1 tsp. baking soda
- 1 tsp. cinnamon

Directions:

1. Grate squash on cheese grater or food processor. Steam in a shallow bowl in microwave with a small amount of water for 3 minutes to soften.
2. Core and grate apple on cheese grater or food processor, and add to squash mixture.
3. Add squash and apple to a mixing bowl and stir in sour cream, egg, and milk with a fork.
4. In a separate bowl, sift flour, baking powder, baking soda, and cinnamon. Add to mixing bowl and stir with the fork.
5. Heat frying pan to low-medium and spray with cooking spray.
6. Using a ladle or a spoon, drop batter onto pan into small pancakes. Flip when bubbles start to form around the edges of pancake.

Apple and Oat Bake

This is a delicious morning treat that is a good source of soluble fiber from the oats and apple that can be helpful for those experiencing diarrhea. Any apple variety would work great for this recipe. Apples are a good source of the phytochemical quercetin, which has antioxidant properties.

Yield: 1 Serving

Ingredients:

- 1 apple
- 1 tsp. cinnamon
- 1/2 tsp. coconut oil
- 1 Tbsp. old-fashioned oats

Directions:

1. Preheat oven to 350°F.
2. Peel and slice apple.
3. Mix apple with cinnamon, 1/2 tsp. coconut oil and old fashioned oats.
4. Place on baking tray.
5. Cover with foil.
6. Bake at 350°F for 20 minutes or until soft.

Nutritional Data: 139 calories, 3 grams fat, 2 grams saturated fat, 0 mg cholesterol, 30.4 grams carbohydrate, 6.1 grams dietary fiber, 1.2 grams protein

Summer Vegetables Omelet

This omelet is an excellent source of protein and includes squash, which is generally a well-tolerated vegetable. Cheddar cheese can be substituted for another flavor of cheese, or lactose-free cheese for those who are lactose intolerant.

Yield: Two 2-egg omelets

Ingredients:

- 2/3 cup sliced summer squash
- 2/3 cup sliced fresh zucchini
- 4 eggs, beaten, divided (may substitute 2 egg whites for each egg if needed for lower fat intake)
- 2 Tbsp. oil, divided
- 2 slices white cheddar cheese (use reduced-fat cheese if experiencing fat intolerance or any flavor cheese of choice)

Directions:

1. Heat 1 Tbsp. oil in omelet pan over medium heat.
2. Sauté zucchini and squash in oil for 4-5 minutes until tender.

3. Remove vegetables and keep warm.
4. Add additional Tbsp. oil to warm pan. Add two beaten eggs and half of the vegetables. Flip and cook thoroughly. Fold in half and top with 1 slice of white cheddar cheese.
5. Make second omelet with remaining ingredients.

Nutritional Data: 310 calories, 27.4 grams fat, 9.1 grams saturated fat, 193 mg cholesterol, 3.6 grams carbohydrate, 0.8 grams dietary fiber, 13.4 grams protein

Lunch and Dinner

Chicken with Quinoa

Prepared as described this recipe will "pack a protein punch," but for additional protein add white beans and cook the quinoa in chicken broth. To add additional flavor or variety, top with low-fat sour cream and salsa for a Mexican-inspired dish. Other grains such as bulgur, rice, or couscous can also be used.

Yield: 6 servings

Ingredients:

- 1 Tbsp. olive oil, divided
- 1 lb. ground chicken breast
- 1 tsp. rosemary
- Pinch salt (optional)
- 1/4 tsp. pepper (optional)
- 1 cup quinoa
- 1 1/2 cups frozen kale
- 1/4 cup chicken broth

Directions:

1. Heat 2 tsp. olive oil in skillet; add the ground chicken, rosemary, salt, and pepper.
2. Cook until cooked through and browned.
3. Add frozen kale and chicken broth and allow to thaw and wilt; approximately 2-3 minutes.
4. While the chicken is cooking, separately cook quinoa according to package directions in medium size saucepan with remaining tsp. of olive oil. Fluff with fork when cooked.
5. Add quinoa to skillet with chicken and kale and combine well. Serve warm.

Nutritional Data: 217 calories, 4.8 grams fat, 0.6 grams saturated fat, 47 mg cholesterol, 19.9 grams carbohydrate, 2.8 grams dietary fiber, 23.9 grams protein

Turkey Meatloaf (Mini)

This healthy alternative to beef meatloaf is adaptable to those dealing with a variety of treatment-related symptom. Providing a generous amount of protein and flavored with vegetables, this meatloaf is sure to satisfy. This is a good selection for those dealing with gastrointestinal upset like nausea or diarrhea, and for those needing blander flavors and less aroma. If you are looking to spice it up, consider adding red pepper flakes, hot sauce, or your favorite BBQ sauce. If looking for a lower-fat alternative, you can use turkey breast meat and add 1/4 cup more broth to this recipe for moistness.

Yield: 8 servings

Ingredients:

- 1 Tbsp. olive oil
- 2 lb. ground turkey (for a leaner preference use 1 lb. breast and 1 lb. dark meat or 2 lb. breast meat for most lean option)
- 1 large or 2 small zucchini
- 2 carrots
- 1/2 medium onion
- 1 cup quick cook oats
- 3/4 cup turkey or chicken broth
- 1 Tbsp. Worcestershire sauce
- 1 Tbsp. ketchup
- 1 egg
- 1 tsp. salt
- 1 tsp. pepper

DIRECTIONS:

Preheat oven to 375°F.

1. Shred zucchini and carrot. Slice onion finely. Alternatively, you can chop ingredients in a mini food processor.
2. Sauté vegetables in olive oil on medium heat until softened, approximately 3 to 4 minutes.
3. While vegetables cook, add broth to oats and let soak.
4. Add cooked vegetables, oats, ketchup, Worcestershire sauce, egg, salt, and pepper to ground turkey.
5. Mix ingredients together, avoid overmixing.
6. Place mixture in a meatloaf shape in a rectangular baking dish and bake for 1 hour until internal thermometer reads at least 165°F. For extra crispy top, broil for the last 5 minutes of cooking, watching closely to avoid burning.

Turkey Tortellini Soup

Many people with pancreatitis do best with simple, comforting meals. This classic soup recipe can be the base for a warm and hearty soup. Yield: 8 Servings

Ingredients:

- 1 12-15 lb. turkey
- 3 medium-size onions
- 6 garlic cloves
- 6 large carrots
- 1 head of celery
- 3 bay leaves
- 6 sprigs fresh thyme
- 1 sprig rosemary
- 3 cups cheese tortellini
- 1 bunch parsley
- 1/2 cup parmigiano cheese
- 1/4 cup extra virgin olive oil

Directions for Roasting the Turkey:

1. Preheat oven to 350°F.
2. Place turkey on roasting rack. Season inside and out with salt and pepper.
3. Roast turkey for 2 1/2 or 3 hours until internal temperature reaches 155°F, basting with natural juices every 30 minutes.
4. Remove turkey and lightly dome with aluminum foil. Allow to cool.

5. Once cool, remove skin and debone turkey.
6. Place body and all bones back into the roasting pan. Roast at 350°F for 30 minutes, until bones are dark, golden brown.
7. Shred turkey meat into bite size pieces.
8. Reserve.

Directions for The Turkey Stock:

1. In a large stock pot, place turkey bones and body, 1/2 head of celery (chopped), 3 carrots (chopped), 2 onions (chopped), 4 garlic cloves (smashed), 3 bay leaves, 1 sprig rosemary and 6 sprigs thyme.
2. Cover with 4 inches of water, bring to a simmer.
3. Lower heat and slowly simmer stock for 2 hours, occasionally skimming fat from the top.
4. After 2 hours, strain stock through a fine sift and cheese cloth.
5. Cool and reserve.

Directions to Assemble the Soup:

1. Add stock to large stock pot.
2. Add all diced vegetables and bring to a simmer. Cook until carrots are tender, approximately 6-8 minutes.

3. Add shredded turkey meat, tortellini, and finely chopped parsley. Adjust soup seasoning with desired amount of kosher salt and fresh ground pepper.

Directions for The Garnish:

1. Remaining celery, small dice (quarter by quarter inch)
2. Remaining carrots, small dice (quarter by quarter inch)
3. Remaining onions, small dice (quarter by quarter inch)
4. Remaining garlic, minced
5. In a large stock pot, put 2 gallons of water. Add 2 Tbsp. of kosher salt. Bring to a rolling boil and add the tortellini.
6. Cook for 6 minutes, occasionally stirring. Strain.
7. Toss 1 Tbsp. extra virgin olive oil into the tortellini.
8. Lay flat on a sheet tray and allow to cool in refrigerator.
9. Reserve.

Nutritional Data: (assumes 1 oz turkey per bowl) 338 calories, 13 grams fat, 3 grams saturated fat, 39 mg cholesterol, 37 grams carbohydrate, 2.5 grams dietary fiber, 19 grams protein.

To Serve

1. In a soup bowl, place 1 large ladle of garnish into center of bowl, top off the bowl with stock.

2. Drizzle with 1/2 tsp. extra virgin olive oil over the top of the soup.
3. Add 1 Tbsp. of grated parmigiano cheese.

Recipe Substitutions:

- If you are not able to tolerate fat in your diet due to fat malabsorption, you can easily substitute the cheese tortellini for plain soup pasta, omit the Parmesan and decrease the amount of oil used.
- For added protein, you can add extra turkey to your soup portion. Each ounce of turkey provides 8 grams of protein.

Shrimp Pomodoro & Angel Hair

This delicious shrimp dish provides a great source of protein, but can be substituted for chicken for those who may be allergic to shellfish. Tomato content can be reduced to a smaller quantity of diced tomato or omitted and replaced with chicken or vegetable broth to reduce acid content. In addition, herbs and spices can be adapted to suit flavor preferences and digestive tolerance. For those looking to add more dietary fiber, whole wheat pasta can be substituted. For those who are experiencing fat malabsorption or dairy intolerance, olive oil can be reduced and parmigiano cheese can be omitted.

Yield: 6 servings

Ingredients:

- 1 lb. angel hair pasta
- 6 Tbsp. extra virgin olive oil
- 3 sprigs fresh thyme
- 8 cloves garlic (sliced paper thin)
- 3/4 cup finely chopped onion
- 1 cup tomato concasse (peeled, seeds removed, diced)
- 1 Tbsp. tomato paste
- 1/2 cup white wine (can substitute non-alcoholic cooking wine)
- 2 Tbsp. chiffonade fresh basil (stacked basil leaves, tightly rolled, thinly sliced)
- 3 Tbsp. crushed red pepper flakes (optional)
- 1 1/2 lb. size 16/20 wild shrimp
- Kosher salt (as needed)
- Fresh ground pepper (as needed)
- 1 Tbsp. minced Italian parsley
- 4 Tbsp. parmigiano cheese (optional)

Directions For Pasta:

1. In a large stock pot add 2 gallons of water and 3 Tbsp. kosher salt; bring to a boil. Add angel hair pasta and boil for 3 minutes, achieving doneness of al dente.
2. Strain pasta and put pasta back into pot. Add 3/4 cup tomato sauce to coat pasta.

Directions for Sauce:

1. In a medium sized sauce pan add 3 Tbsp. of extra virgin olive oil over medium heat and add onions. Sweat onions for 5 minutes until translucent, then add half the amount of garlic, red pepper flakes (if wanted), 2 sprigs of thyme and tomato paste.
2. Continue to cook over medium heat for 3 minutes. Add white wine (reserving 1 Tbsp. for shrimp).
3. Continue to stir and cook until wine is evaporated. Add tomato concasse, 1 tsp. kosher salt and desired amount of fresh ground pepper. Lower heat to slow simmer for 45 minutes.
4. After 45 minutes, with a hand blender, pulse to slightly puree (you do not want the sauce to be completely smooth). Pulses should be 15 2-second pulses.
5. Add parsley. Reserve for plating.

Method for Assembly:

1. Heat shrimp in remaining tomato sauce. Place desired amount of pasta into a pasta bowl.
2. Spoon over tomato sauce. Add desired amount of shrimp and fresh basil. Each dish can be garnished with 1 Tbsp. parmigiano cheese.

Directions for Shrimp:

1. In a medium sauté pan that's been pre-heated over medium-high heat, add the remaining olive oil and garlic.
2. When the garlic begins to slightly brown, add shrimp that has been shelled and de-veined, season with salt and pepper. Sauté for 1-2 minutes over high heat.
3. Add remaining fresh thyme and 1 Tbsp of white wine. Remove from heat.
4. Reserve for plate assembly.

Recipe Note: Will have zero alcohol content when cooked. For those who want to remove the alcohol completely can do so.

Recipe is easily adaptable for different tastes or for what someone can tolerate.

Nutritional Data: 497 calories, 17.8 grams fat, 3.4 grams saturated fat, 189 mg cholesterol, 49.3 grams carbohydrate, 1.8 grams dietary fiber, 34 grams protein

Asparagus Frittata

Frittatas are very versatile – they can be used at any meal as a main dish, side dish or appetizer, and can easily be turned into a quiche by adding a pie crust at the bottom (if able to tolerate higher amounts of fat). Eggs provide the highest quality protein available in any food. This recipe is great for those needing easy-to-chew/swallow foods.

Yield: 1 - 9-inch quiche, serves 6

Ingredients:

- 1/2 lb. fresh asparagus, trimmed and cut into 1/2-inch pieces
- 1 egg white, lightly beaten
- 4 eggs, beaten
- 1/4 tsp. ground nutmeg
- 1 Tbsp. Dijon mustard
- 1 cup shredded Swiss or muenster cheese (use reduced-fat cheese if experiencing fat intolerance)

- Salt and pepper to taste

Directions:

1. Preheat oven to 375°F.
2. Add asparagus to saucepan with 1 inch of water or place in a steamer. Steam for 4-6 minutes or until tender, but not mushy. Once steamed, allow it to drain well and cool.
3. Coat pie dish with nonstick cooking spray.
4. Add drained and dried asparagus to pie dish.
5. In a bowl, beat together eggs, milk, mustard, nutmeg, salt and pepper. Add shredded cheese and mix in.
6. Pour egg mixture into pie pan.
7. Bake uncovered in preheated oven until firm, about 40-50 minutes.
8. Enjoy warm or at room temperature.

Nutritional Data: 173 calories, 7.2 grams fat, 1 gram saturated fat, 50 mg cholesterol, 3.6 grams carbohydrate, 1 gram dietary fiber, 24.3 grams protein

Edamame Hummus Wrap

Soy is a high-quality protein that does not cause the same discomfort as other beans and hummuses. This recipe is extremely easy and satisfying. It can be delicious plain or with any added vegetables that you can tolerate (those with diarrhea or indigestion should be sure to use well-cooked vegetables without the skin).

Yield: 4 servings

Ingredients:

- 1 cup cooked shelled edamame
- 1/4 cup Tahini (sesame paste)
- 1 Tbsp. lemon juice
- Garlic clove, peeled
- 2 Tbsp. coarsely chopped fresh herbs (such as rosemary, thyme, and basil)
- 2 Tbsp. olive oil
- Salt to taste (approximately 1/4 tsp.)
- 4 flour wraps
- Optional: Sautéed or roasted vegetables, or fresh, raw vegetables that you can tolerate

Directions:

1. Combine edamame, Tahini, lemon juice, garlic, and herbs in food processor.
2. Process ingredients until smooth.
3. Drizzle olive oil through feed tube of food processor, continuing to process until the oil is fully incorporated into the hummus mixture.
4. Season with salt to taste.
5. Spread 1/4 cup hummus in each wrap, top with raw or roasted vegetables of choice, roll and serve.

Nutritional Data: 399 calories, 21.9 grams fat, 3.1 grams saturated fat, 0 mg cholesterol, 39.9 grams carbohydrate, 4.1 grams dietary fiber, 12.1 grams protein

Chicken Salad Sandwich

This sandwich is very easy to prepare and contains satisfying flavors and textures. It is a well-balanced meal that includes protein and carbohydrates, along with a splash of colorful fruit and herbs. For those experiencing fat intolerance, reduced-fat mayo can be substituted and walnuts can be avoided. You also can experiment with other herbs like rosemary or basil for varied flavors.

Yield: 4 sandwiches

Ingredients:

- 2 chicken breasts (skin on during cooking only) or approximately 2 cups diced or shredded cooked, skinless chicken
- 2 Tbsp. mayonnaise (may substitute yogurt - low fat or Greek - and 1 tsp. lemon juice)
- 1/4 cup sliced grapes
- 2 Tbsp. dried cranberries
- 1/4 cup chopped walnuts (optional)
- 2 tsp. dried tarragon
- 8 slices bread

Directions:

1. Preheat oven to 375°F.
2. Roast chicken breasts for approximately 45 minutes until cooked through, juices run clear and temperature of chicken reaches 165°F.
3. Remove skin from breast meat. Discard skin. Cube, dice, or shred meat.

4. Add mayonnaise, grapes, cranberries, walnuts, and tarragon.
5. Mix well and divide into 4 (~3/4 cup) portions and spread onto bread. Delicious with toasted bread!

Nutritional Data: 237 calories, 9.8 grams fat, 1.4 grams saturated fat, 56 mg cholesterol, 13.1 grams carbohydrate, 1.2 grams dietary fiber, 23.7 grams protein

Hearty Vegetable and Lentil Soup

This hearty soup is very versatile and can be adapted for whatever vegetables you have available. Use this dish as a complement to a meal or serve with homemade corn bread to complete a meal. The vegetables and lentils provide an excellent amount of insoluble and soluble fiber, and this dish is a great choice for those dealing with constipation.

Yield: 6 servings

Ingredients:

- 3 cups water
- 3 cups vegetable or chicken broth

- 3 medium carrots, chopped
- 1 medium onion, chopped
- 1 cup dried lentils, rinsed
- 2 celery ribs, sliced
- 1 small bell pepper, color of your choice
- 1/4 cup uncooked brown rice
- 1 tsp. dried basil or 1 Tbsp. of fresh chopped basil
- 1 garlic clove, minced
- 1 bay leaf
- 1/2 cup tomato paste

Directions:

1. In a large saucepan, combine all ingredients except tomato paste. Bring to a boil.
2. Reduce heat; cover and simmer for 1 to 1 1/2 hours or until lentils and rice are tender.
3. Add the tomato paste and stir until blended. Cook for 10-15 minutes. Discard bay leaf.

Nutritional Data: 206 calories, 1.4 grams fat, 0 grams saturated fat, 0 mg cholesterol, 36 grams carbohydrate, 12.6 grams dietary fiber, 12.9 grams protein

Pastiera (Pasta Egg Bake)

Pastiera is traditionally an Italian-style Easter cake that is sweetened and made with ricotta cheese. This recipe is a savory spin on this classic dish and is packed with protein from the eggs and milk. Lactose-free milk and cheese can be used for those experiencing lactose intolerance. Spaghetti squash also is a great substitution for pasta noodles as a lower carbohydrate alternative or for those looking to add a tolerable vegetable component.

Yield: 8 servings

Ingredients:

- 12 eggs, beaten (may substitute for lower fat pasteurized liquid egg product)
- 2 cups of milk (substitute non-fat or reduced-fat milk if experiencing fat intolerance)
- Salt and pepper to taste
- 1 cup of grated Parmesan cheese
- Perciatelli (aka Bucatini or macaroni spaghetti with a hole running through)

Directions:

1. Preheat oven to 250°F. Spray a rectangular 9"x13" baking dish with nonfat cooking spray.
2. Cook pasta according to package directions.
3. Mix beaten eggs with milk, salt, pepper, and cheese while macaroni is cooking.
4. Combine together in the 9"x13" baking dish.
5. Bake at 250°F for 10 minutes, and then increase oven temperature to 350°F for 25-30 minutes.
6. Cut into 8 pieces, or smaller as a side dish.

Nutritional Data: 378 calories, 11.5 grams fat, 4.6 grams saturated fat, 259 mg cholesterol, 48.5 grams carbohydrate, 2 grams dietary fiber, 21.4 grams protein

Apps & Sides

Maple Green Beans

Roasting green beans is a quick and easy way to prepare a delicious green vegetable. This recipe can be made with fresh out-of-the-garden green beans, fresh packaged and pre-washed green beans, or frozen green beans. Boost the flavor by using pure maple syrup.

Yield: 4 servings

Ingredients:

- 1 lb. green beans
- 1 Tbsp. maple syrup
- 1 tsp. olive oil
- 1/2 tsp. salt
- 1/4 tsp. pepper

Directions:

1. Preheat oven to 400°F.
2. In a large bowl, toss green beans with maple syrup, oil, salt and pepper.
3. Arrange evenly on sheet tray.

4. Roast until tender, about 20 to 25 minutes.

Nutritional Data: 59 calories, 1.3 grams fat, 0 grams saturated fat, 0 mg cholesterol, 11.5 grams carbohydrate, 3.9 grams dietary fiber, 2.1 grams protein

Carrot Purée with Olive Oil and Cilantro

This is the perfect side dish for the holiday season, especially for patients facing pancreatitis, as it is a well-cooked vegetable dish that is easier to digest and less likely to aggravate digestive issues. The carrots provide an excellent source of beta-carotene. The oil may be reduced if sensitive to fat, or coconut oil may be substituted (which may be more easily absorbed). If you are sensitive to additional herbed flavors, the cilantro can be reduced or omitted. This purée can also translate well to any other root vegetable or squash such as turnip, parsnip, acorn squash, or butternut squash.

Yield: 6 servings

Ingredients:

- About 10 carrots, peeled and cubed

- 5 Tbsp. extra virgin olive oil
- Sea salt
- Fresh black pepper
- 3 Tbsp. finely chopped fresh cilantro (may substitute other fresh herbs of choice and as tolerated)

Directions:

1. In a large pot, boil peeled and cubed carrots for about 20 minutes until they are very tender. (Alternatively, steaming them in a steam pan over boiling water may preserve the maximum amount of nutrients.)
2. In a medium pan, add fresh cilantro leaves and 3 Tbsp. of extra virgin olive oil. Heat on lowest flame for about 5 minutes.
3. Remove from heat and allow to sit for about 5 minutes. Remove cilantro from oil and set aside.
4. In a food processor or using an immersion blender, add in cooked carrots and cilantro oil and 2 Tbsp. of extra virgin olive oil. Purée until smooth.
5. Add sea salt and fresh black pepper to taste and fresh cilantro as a garnish.

Nutritional Data: 142 calories, 11.7 grams fat, 1.7 grams saturated fat, 0 mg cholesterol, 10 grams carbohydrate, 2.5 grams dietary fiber, 0.8 grams protein

Vegetable Popover

These vegetable popovers are excellent for individuals needing soft, easy-to-swallow foods. Eggs (or egg substitute) add an excellent source of high-quality protein. This also is a great recipe to prepare ahead of time and reheat as a healthy mini-meal.

Yield: 6 servings

Ingredients:

- 1 zucchini, chopped into bite-size pieces
- 1 large carrot, chopped into small pieces (about half the size of the zucchini)
- 2 tsp. olive oil
- 6 large eggs
- 1/4 cup milk (non-dairy alternative, if desired)
- 1/3 cup shredded cheddar cheese (use reduced-fat cheese for those experiencing fat intolerance)

- Salt and freshly ground black pepper, to taste
- Pinch of turmeric
- Onion powder, to taste

Directions:

1. Preheat the oven to 350°F.
2. Spray 6 muffin cups with nonstick spray.
3. Sauté the zucchini and the carrots in 2 tsp. olive oil for 5-7 minutes.
4. In a medium bowl, whisk together the eggs and milk. Add salt, pepper, turmeric, and onion powder.
5. Distribute egg mixture evenly into muffin cups.
6. Distribute zucchini and carrots into egg mixture.
7. Bake 25 to 30 minutes, or until egg is cooked through.

Nutritional Data: 126 calories, 8.9 grams fat, 3.2 grams saturated fat, 193 mg cholesterol, 3.4 grams carbohydrate, 0.7 grams dietary fiber, 8.7 grams protein

Butternut Squash Soup

Enjoy this colorful, smooth soup as a great complement to any entrée or as a main dish. Use prepared, frozen, fresh squash, or canned pumpkin to reduce the preparation time. This soup is a good choice for those looking for a low-fat, simple meal option. This also is a great soup to make in a large batch and freeze extra portions. Yield: 8 servings

Ingredients:

- 1 large butternut squash (or 2 lb. frozen cubed or two 16 oz. cans pumpkin)
- 3 carrots, roughly chopped
- 2 stalk celery, roughly chopped
- 1/2 medium onion, roughly chopped
- 2 Tbsp. olive oil
- 4 cups chicken stock
- Salt and pepper to taste
- 1 Tbsp. cinnamon

Directions:

1. Preheat oven to 400°F.
2. Clean and halve squash lengthwise and remove seeds.

3. Drizzle 1 Tbsp. olive oil on squash and place face down on baking sheet.
4. Roast squash until tender, approximately 25 minutes. Remove from oven to cool.
5. While roasting, sauté vegetables in stock pot in 1 Tbsp. olive oil.
6. Once squash cools, scoop out flesh and add to pot with chicken stock.
7. Add cinnamon.
8. Cook for approximately 5 minutes on medium heat.
9. Use immersion blender (or transfer to blender) to purée soup; cook an additional 3-5 minutes.

Nutritional Data: 100 calories, 3.9 grams fat, 0.6 grams saturated fat, 0 mg cholesterol, 17.2 grams carbohydrate, 3.5 grams dietary fiber, 1.8 grams protein 48

Holiday & Seasonal Ideas

Chicken Kebab with Tzatziki and Pita

A great summertime chicken recipe topped with cool, creamy tzatziki sauce. Preparation is required 2-3 hours ahead of time but well worth the extra wait time. Choose this recipe for those needing high protein, low fiber choices.

Yield: 6 servings

Ingredients:

Pita:

- 1 pack store-bought pita bread

Tzatziki sauce:

- 3 cucumbers
- 12 oz. plain Greek yogurt
- 1 pinch of sea salt
- 1/2 tsp. extra virgin olive oil
- 2 cloves of garlic, minced

Chicken:

- 1 1/2 pounds skinless, boneless chicken breast halves, cut into 1/2-inch pieces
- 1/4 cup olive oil for marinade
- 2 Tbsp. lemon juice
- 1 tsp. dried oregano
- 1/2 tsp. sea salt
- 6 wooden skewers

Directions for Tzatsiki Sauce:

1. Clean and grate cucumbers. Be sure to remove seeds and peel off cucumber skin if on a low-fiber diet.
2. Strain juice and place in medium bowl.
3. Add yogurt to bowl and mix cucumbers, garlic, salt and olive oil together.
4. Cover and refrigerate for 30 minutes.

Directions for Chicken and Pita:

1. Combine 1/4 cup olive oil, lemon juice, 1 tsp. oregano, and 1/2 tsp. sea salt in a large bowl.
2. Add chicken, mix with the marinade and cover the bowl.
3. Marinate in the refrigerator for at least 2 hours.

4. Skewer chicken evenly on 6 wooden skewers. Preheat grill, place pitas on grill for 2 minutes on each side until slightly browned.
5. Remove from grill and set aside.
6. Cook the skewers on the preheated grill, turning frequently until nicely browned on all sides, about 10 minutes per side. Serve with 57 grilled pita and topped with tzatziki sauce.

Nutritional Data: 441 calories, 13.8 grams fat, 3 grams saturated fat, 67 mg cholesterol, 44.7 grams carbohydrate, 3 grams dietary fiber, 34.9 grams protein

Pumpkin Oatmeal Bars

These are a healthy alternative to many common cookie recipes. Whole-wheat flour, oats, pumpkin and ground flaxseed add soluble and insoluble fiber, along with the phytochemical and antioxidant benefits of the added spices. Great selections for an after-dinner dessert or midday snack. Flaxseed can be omitted if experiencing gas, bloating, or diarrhea.

Yield: 40 square bars or 48 cookies

Ingredients:

- 2 cups whole-wheat flour
- 1 1/3 cups rolled oats
- 1 tsp. baking soda
- 3/4 tsp. salt
- 1 tsp. cinnamon
- 1/2 tsp. nutmeg
- 1 1/3 cup sugar
- 2/3 cup canola oil
- 3 Tbsp. molasses
- 1 can of cooked pumpkin puree
- 1 tsp. vanilla
- 2 Tbsp. ground flaxseed (optional)
- Optional add-ins: 1 cup mini chocolate chips

Directions:

1. Preheat oven to 350°F. Grease two 12"x17" baking sheet pans.
2. Mix together flour, oats, baking soda, salt, and spices.
3. In a separate bowl, mix together sugar, oil, molasses, pumpkin, vanilla, and optional flaxseeds until very well combined.

4. Mix flour and sugar mixtures together. Fold in chocolate chips, if desired.
5. Spread and press batter onto greased cookie sheets (to make cookies, drop 1 inch size balls of batter an inch apart, and flatten tops of cookies with fork or your fingers to press into cookie shape).
6. Bake for 16 minutes or until inserted knife or toothpick is clean. Rotate halfway through baking.
7. Remove from oven (if making cookies, transfer to wire rack to cool).
8. Once cool slice into 20 bars per sheet pan.

Nutritional Data: 101 calories, 4 grams fat, 0 grams saturated fat, 0 mg cholesterol, 15.4 grams carbohydrate, 0.9 grams dietary fiber, 1.2 grams protein

Sweet Potato and White Bean Fritters

Trying this unique plant-based recipe will add vibrancy and texture to your plate. Substitute any squash or beans that you have available. This recipe is a good choice for those needing foods that are soft and easy to chew and swallow.

Yield: 12 fritters

Ingredients:

- 2 cups (10 oz.) cubed and peeled sweet potato
- 1 can (15.5 oz.) no-added salt white beans, drained and rinsed
- 4 Tbsp. quick cooking oats
- 1 large egg
- 1/4 cup onion, minced
- 1 large clove garlic, minced
- 2 tsp. chopped fresh sage leaves
- 1/4 tsp. cumin
- Salt and freshly ground pepper to taste
- 1 Tbsp. canola oil or extra virgin olive oil, divided
- 3/4 cup low-fat sour cream or fat-free plain Greek-style yogurt

Directions:

1. In large saucepan with a steamer basket, steam sweet potatoes until tender, about 15-17 minutes.
2. Transfer sweet potato to food processor. Add beans, oats, egg, onion, garlic, sage, cumin. Pulse until blended yet slightly chunky.
3. Season with salt and pepper.
4. Heat 1 Tbsp. oil in large skillet over medium-high heat.
5. Gently drop six 1/4 cup portions of mixture into pan and gently press into round patties with back of measuring cup or spatula. Don't over crowd skillet.
6. Sauté fritters until golden brown on bottom, about 5 minutes. Heat may need to be adjusted for optimal browning.
7. Carefully turn over each fritter and sauté until other side is golden brown, about 3-4 minutes.
8. Transfer fritters to plate and cover with foil to keep warm.
9. Use remaining oil to sauté remaining six fritters. There should be 12 fritters in total. Serve 61 warm with sour cream or Greek yogurt.

Nutritional Data: 104 calories, 4.9 grams fat, 2.1 grams saturated fat, 22 mg cholesterol, 12.5 grams carbohydrate, 2.7 grams dietary fiber, 3.7 grams protein

Thanksgiving Meatballs

This is a unique twist to a comfort food that takes meatballs from savory to slightly sweet. It's a great choice for those needing low-fat protein choices during the holiday. Yield: 16 medium-sized meatballs, 8 servings

Ingredients:

- 1 1/2 lb. ground turkey meat (you can use half ground turkey and half sweet turkey sausage for extra flavor)
- 1 1/4 cup of herbed stuffing bread cubes
- 1/2 cup dried cranberries
- 1 large egg plus 1 egg white
- 1/4 cup finely chopped sweet onion
- 1 Tbsp. chopped fresh sage
- 1 tsp. salt
- 1 Tbsp. olive oil

- Other add-in ideas: shredded carrots or chopped mushrooms

Directions:

1. Preheat oven to 450°F.
2. Coat a 9"x13" inch baking sheet with olive oil and set aside.
3. In a large bowl, combine the ground turkey/turkey sausage, cranberries, eggs, onion, sage, and salt. Add half of the stuffing cubes in whole form, and crush the other half in your hands to resemble bread crumbs. Mix everything together with your hands until it is all incorporated.
4. Coat your hands with a little bit of olive oil and roll the mixture firmly into balls about the size of golf balls. Place the meatballs in the baking dish directly next to each other in rows. This will help them keep their shape while baking.
5. Roast for about 20 minutes, until the meatballs are cooked through and slightly brown on top.
6. Serve meatballs with gravy and cranberry sauce, and enjoy!

Nutritional Data: 192 calories, 7.9 grams fat, 1.8 grams saturated fat, 73 mg cholesterol, 5.4 grams carbohydrate, 0.9 grams dietary fiber, 18.5 grams protein

Sole En Papillote with Citrus and Ginger

This delicately flavored Sole recipe provides an excellent source of protein and healthy fats. This recipe is great for those who need lighter flavors and less fiber.

For those more sensitive, the quantity of onion, garlic, and ginger can be reduced as needed.

Yield: 4 servings

Ingredients:

- Parchment paper
- 4 sole fillets (6 oz. each)
- 2 Tbsp. olive oil
- 3 cloves garlic, diced
- 4 scallions, sliced
- 2 Tbsp. peeled, minced ginger root
- 2 Tbsp. grated orange rind

- 1/4-inch thick circular slices from 2 medium oranges
- 1/2 tsp. kosher salt
- 1/4 tsp. freshly ground black pepper

Directions:

1. Heat oven to 450°F.
2. Fold four 15 inch square pieces of parchment paper in half. Starting at fold of each piece, draw half a large heart shape. Cut along lines; open. Place 1 fish fillet next to crease on each piece of parchment.
3. In a small skillet, heat 1 1/2 Tbsp. oil over medium heat. Sauté sliced garlic, scallions, ginger root and orange rind for approximately 1 minute (until garlic golden). Remove skillet from heat.
4. Sprinkle fish fillets with salt and pepper. Divide mixture from skillet among fish. Top each fish with orange "circles." Fold other half of parchment over fish. Starting at top of each parchment half heart, make small, tight, overlapping folds along outside edge to seal packet; twist tail ends to seal.
5. Place packets on rimmed baking sheet and roast for 8-10 minutes.

Nutritional Data: 303 calories, 9.7 grams fat, 1.6 grams saturated fat, 116 mg cholesterol, 10.8 grams carbohydrate, 2.4 grams dietary fiber, 42.2 grams protein

Vegan Tofu Lasagna

This is a great alternative for those foregoing animal-based products or looking to cut back on added fats. Tofu, from soybeans, provides an excellent amount of high quality protein, phytochemicals and fiber. Great recipe for diets requiring lower fat content or ingredients that are easy to chew/swallow. For those sensitive to tomato sauce, you can use olive oil to coat dish and make lasagna roll-ups with tofu mixture and sautéed vegetables like zucchini, squash, carrot and mushrooms.

Yield: 8 servings

Ingredients:

- 2 Tbsp. olive oil
- 1/2 tsp. salt
- 1 tsp. Italian seasoning
- 16 oz. extra firm tofu

- 2 cloves garlic (or 1 tsp. powdered garlic)
- 1 Tbsp. nutritional yeast
- 10 oz. frozen kale (or spinach, collards), defrosted, water extracted
- 1 package lasagna noodles
- 16 oz. tomato sauce

Directions:

1. Preheat oven to 350°F.
2. Drain the tofu and pat dry with paper towels.
3. Crumble into the bowl of a food processor or high-speed blender.
4. Add Italian seasoning, garlic and nutritional yeast.
5. Process on high until smooth and "ricotta-like."
6. Add the defrosted kale to the blended tofu mixture.
7. Cook lasagna noodles according to package directions until al dente. Drain and cool.
8. Pour about 1/2 cup pasta sauce into the bottom of a 9"x13" baking or lasagna pan.
9. Layer noodles with tofu mixture and a few spoonfuls of sauce until you reach three layers.
10. Smother with remaining tomato sauce.

11. Bake for approximately 30 minutes until sauce is bubbly and lasagna is heated through.

Nutritional Data: 262 calories, 7.1 grams fat, 1 gram saturated fat, 19 mg cholesterol, 37.8 grams carbohydrate, 2.5 grams dietary fiber, 13.5 grams protein

Turkey Sweet Potato Hash

Since fatigue is sometimes experienced by people living with pancreatitis, this easy-to-prepare dish is nutrient dense and a good source of protein and B vitamins, which can help boost energy. In addition, the cooked apple and sweet potato provide fiber that is easily tolerated and full of antioxidants like betacarotene and quercetin. The ingredients include a variety of appealing textures and flavors of the holiday season!

Yield: 6 servings

Ingredients:

- 2 medium sweet potatoes, peeled and cut into 1/2-inch pieces

- 1 medium apple, cored and cut into 1/2 -inch pieces (Honeycrisp or Braeburn work wonderfully, although any apple can suit this recipe)
- 1/2 cup reduced-fat sour cream (may also substitute reduced-fat yogurt)
- 1 tsp. lemon juice
- 1 Tbsp. olive oil
- 1 medium shallot, chopped
- 3 cups diced, cooked, skinless turkey breast (or chicken)
- 1 tsp. dried rosemary (1 Tbsp. fresh, chopped)
- Salt and pepper, to taste

Directions:

1. Place sweet potatoes in a steamer basket and cook for approximately 10 minutes. Add apple and cook until everything is just tender, about 3 minutes longer. Be sure that they are not overly mushy. Drain and set aside.
2. Transfer 1 cup of the mixture to a large bowl; mash. Stir in sour cream and lemon juice. Add the remaining sweet potato/apple mixture and stir gently to mix.

3. Heat oil in a large skillet over medium-high heat. Add shallot until softened, 1 to 2 minutes. Add turkey (or chicken), rosemary, salt and pepper.
4. Stir mixture occasionally and cook until heated through, about 2 minutes.
5. Add the reserved sweet potato/apple mixture to the pan. Press on the hash with a wide metal spoon or spatula. Cook hash until the bottom is lightly browned, about 3 minutes.
6. Divide into multiple sections with spatula; flip and cook until the bottom sides are browned, about 2 to 3 minutes.
7. Serve promptly.

Desserts & Beverages

Rice Pudding

A creamy, often well-tolerated, high-calorie pudding that works as a great dessert for those needing to add protein and calories to their daily intake. For those requiring a lower fat alternative, reduced-fat milk may be substituted. Non-dairy, lactose-free options like soy, rice, or almond milk can work as well.

Yield: 4 servings

Ingredients:

- 2 cups of whole milk, reduced-fat milk, or non-dairy alternative
- 1/3 cup of sugar
- 3/4 cups of long grain white or brown rice
- 1/4 tsp. salt
- 1 egg (beaten)
- 1/2 tsp. vanilla extract
- 1/4 cup dried fruit of your choice (optional)
- Cinnamon or nutmeg for sprinkling on top (optional)

- Tip: for extra cinnamon flavor, boil rice with a cinnamon stick added to the water

Directions:

1. First rinse uncooked rice with cold water.
2. Bring 1 1/2 cups of water to a boil.
3. Add rice, reduce heat, and cook for approximately 20 minutes until tender.
4. In large pot add rice, 1 1/2 cups milk, sugar and salt.
5. Stir rice constantly to avoid rice from sticking to bottom of pot.
6. Cook until mixture is a thick and creamy texture, approximately 20 minutes.
7. Remove pot from heat, and while still hot, add remaining 1/2 cup milk, beaten eggs (add very slowly while stirring pot), vanilla, and optional dried fruit (such as raisins).
8. Return to medium heat and stir again until slightly thickened (5-10 minutes max).
9. Remove from heat, and pour into containers. Top with a sprinkling of cinnamon or nutmeg for garnish as desired.
10. Refrigerate before serving.

Nutritional Data: 289 calories, 5.9 grams fat, 0.5 grams saturated fat, 59 mg cholesterol, 50 grams carbohydrate, 51 1.2 grams dietary fiber, 8.1 grams protein

Peaches and Cream Smoothie

Simple meals like shakes and smoothies are often helpful ways for people caring for or living with pancreatitis to get the nutrients they need. This Peaches and Cream Smoothie combines the potassium and fiber benefits of peaches and bananas along with soluble fiber from rolled oats, which can help to alleviate loose bowel movements and promote regularity. The protein powder can be added at the recommendation of your healthcare team for additional nutritional value. Dairy components can be easily substituted with lactose-free or non-dairy versions. Yield: 1-2 servings

Ingredients:

- 1/2 cup rolled oats
- 1/3 cup plain yogurt (or soy coconut/almond yogurt)
- 3/4 cup milk (or soy/almond/rice milk) + 1/4 cup more for morning

- • 1 small ripe peach (or 1/2 cup frozen peaches, thawed and softened)
- 1/2 medium banana
- Pinch of salt
- 1-2 Tbsp. protein powder (whey or soy) (optional)

Directions:

1. Gather all ingredients.

2. Combine ingredients in a blender and enjoy.

3. Store in a container in your refrigerator overnight if making ahead of time. In the morning, add last 1/4 cup of milk, more if you need it to blend smoothly.

Nutritional Data: (assumes regular whole milk and yogurt) 426 calories, 9 grams fat, 4.5 grams saturated fat, 25 mg cholesterol, 68 grams carbohydrate, 7 grams dietary fiber, 20 grams protein

Grilled Pineapple

A superb dessert to make when you already have the grill going, this low-calorie, low- fat treat is easy and impressive.

Yield: Serves 4

Ingredients

- 1 tablespoon unsalted butter 2 teaspoons brown sugar Juice of ½ lime
- 1 fresh pineapple, cored and cut into eighths, lengthwise

Directions

1. Place the butter, brown sugar and lime juice in a small bowl and mix well. Prepare a grill or preheat the broiler.
2. Brush butter mixture on the pineapple, place on the grill or under the broiler and cook, turning once, until lightly browned on both sides, about 4 minutes.
3. Drizzle with the remaining butter mixture.

Nutritional Data: Calories 142, Total Fat 3g, Saturated Fat 1g, Trans Fat 0g, Cholesterol 3mg, Sodium 4mg, Total Carbohydrate 21g, Dietary Fiber 3g, Protein 1g

Banana Peach Sorbet

You don't need an ice cream machine to make this incredibly easy and quick dessert. You do, however, need to keep an arsenal of frozen fruit in the freezer. You can substitute the peaches with any kind of berry, mangoes, papayas or simply add more bananas, or jazz it up with ground cinnamon or nutmeg. For those who want something a little sweeter, swirl in any flavor of unsweetened fruit spread.

Yield: Serves 4

Ingredients

1. 2 over - ripe bananas, thinly sliced and frozen
2. 2 cups chopped fresh peaches, peeled, if desired and frozen
3. ½ teaspoon vanilla extract 1/3 cup plain low-fat yogurt
4. Place the frozen bananas and peaches in the bowl of a food processor fitted with a steel blade. Process until smooth. Gradually add the vanilla and yogurt and process until completely incorporated. Serve immediately.

Nutritional Data: Calories 93, Total Fat 1g, Saturated Fat 0g, Trans Fat 0g, Cholesterol 1mg, Sodium 15mg, Total Carbohydrate 22g, Dietary Fiber 3g, Protein 14g

Baked Apples

Tart, sweet, warm and comforting, these apples can be served hot, cold or at room temperature. Feel free to use any variety of apple you like.

Yield: Serves 4

Ingredients

- 1 tablespoon maple syrup
- 1/2 teaspoon ground cinnamon 1/4 cup raisins or currants
- 1/3 cup orange juice
- 2 strips lemon zest, grated or chopped (optional)
- 4 Granny Smith apples, cored and top third cut off and discarded

Directions

1. Preheat the oven to 375 degrees.

2. Place the maple syrup, cinnamon, raisins and, if desired, the lemon peel, in a small bowl and mix well. Place apples in a small baking dish, so that they touch each other. Divide the maple syrup mixture into four parts and stuff inside apples. Pour the orange juice around them.
3. Transfer to the oven and bake until the apples are soft, about one hour.

Nutritional Data: Calories 140, Total Fat 0g, Saturated Fat 0g, Trans Fat 0g, Cholesterol 0mg, Sodium 3mg, Total Carbohydrate 37g, Dietary Fiber 6g, Protein 1g

The Bottom Line

Pancreatitis is an inflammation of the pancreas and can be both acute or chronic. When the pancreas is inflamed, the main functions of digesting food and producing insulin can be impaired.

To manage pancreatitis, a special diet should be followed. A pancreatitis diet generally includes plenty of fruits and vegetables, whole grains, and lean proteins.

Foods high in fat and sugar should be kept to a minimum. Medications such as pancreatic enzymes and supplements such as MCT oil are sometimes used to assist with symptoms.

Following the pancreatitis diet will help prevent further damage to the pancreas, manage symptoms, and avoid malnutrition.

Made in the USA
Las Vegas, NV
27 February 2021